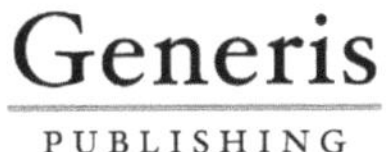

Comparative differential study of comorbid symptomatic groups

associated with Autism Spectrum Disorder diagnosis

Manuel Ojea Rúa
Tania Justo Román
Lydia Castro Núñez

Title: **Comparative differential study of comorbid symptomatic groups**

associated with Autism Spectrum Disorder diagnosis

ISBN: 979-8-89248-450-3

Author: Manuel Ojea Rúa, Tania Justo Román,Lydia Castro Núñez

Cover image: https://pixabay.com/

Publisher: Generis Publishing
Online orders: www.generis-publishing.com
Contact email: info@generis-publishing.com

Comparative differential study of comorbid symptomatic groups associated with Autism Spectrum Disorder diagnosis

Manuel Ojea Rúa (PhD. Pyschology. University of Vigo)

Lydia Castro Núñez (MEd Biology.University of Vigo)

Lourdes Rivas Otero (MEd Psyco-pedagogy. University of Vigo)

Tania Justo Román (MEd Music- therapy.University of Vigo)

Social Institute of Scientific Research on Autism Spectrum Disorder.

TIC: G-44568509

Address: Faculty of Education Sciences (University of Vigo).

Mail: lictea2@gmail.com

Mail: moxea@uvigo.es

Availability of materials

All data to this study are realised throughout the year 2022-23.

Declaration of conflicting interests

Authors declared no potential conflicts of interest with respect to the research, authorship, and/or publication of this article.

ORCID iD

Manuel Ojea: https://orcid.org/my-orcid?orcid=0000-0002-9787-2520

Abstract

Individuals with autism spectrum disorders (ASD) make up a diagnosis characterized by a multifunctional neurocognitive disorder, based on a limited structure to perform nodal-synaptic interrelationships between the contents of learning. Likewise, this disorder may be associated with a set of comorbid symptom groups, which, regarding their intensity, may border with ASD main diagnosis and lead to basic errors that affect subsequent social- educational treatment. This study analyses most recurrent associated comorbid groups, as well as, if the presence of symptomatic comorbid groups is differential regarding group shape: normotypical and ASD groups. A total of 390 children participated in this study, 128 belonged to normotypical group and 262 did it to experimental group, subdivided into three levels of ASD. Results found through multivariate- test indicate that the whole dimension significantly affects group way intersection, age and sex (sig: .00). The post-hoc test analysis indicates this influence was differential regarding to the group type for the following dimensions: cognition, behaviour, psychoaffectivity, language and psychomotor disorder, while relative differences were not observed in specific- clinical dimension, where only epilepsy showed a differential result: no differences were found in general- clinic dimension.

Lay abstract

ASD′ diagnosis and treatment shows, to date, many weak points that need to be improved. Previous studies have shown how important is the psycho-educational component regarding ASD treatment, therefore it is necessary to understand the specific characteristics of the nuclear ASD diagnosis, in order to work out a specific therapy according to every single case.

In the current study, we examined and analysed ASD patients as well as participants showing comorbid symptoms such as epilepsy, in order to show how these comorbidities can reach a very high level, leading to a confused and wrong ASD nuclear diagnosis.

Therefore, it is essential to gain more insight into the specific diagnosis process, defining the ASD symptoms very precisely in order to develop more accurate and specific educational programs.

This study contributes to the improvement in ASD diagnosis, providing a large number of participants in order to study the relation between several comorbid symptoms and its reliability as ASD indicative factors or not.

Keywords

Autism Spectrum Disorder, Comorbidity, diagnosis, synapse- neural- nodes.

TABLE OF CONTENTS

Introduction

Ojea (2021) defined ASD as a multifactorial neurodevelopmental disorder, characterized by presence of heterogeneous behaviour in addition to behavioural indications of International Classification "DSM-5" (APA, 2013). In his experimental study to N: 121, it the presence of a multivariate set of symptoms associated co-occurring with ASD, which make up the associated constant symptomatic comorbidity, which is not isolated element of this diagnosis, but ASD diagnosis co-occurs with a set of permanently associated clinical symptoms. Indeed, these considerations are very important, since the disorder could often be situated within the limits of very subtle distal proximity with its associated symptomatic comorbidity, which can lead to obvious errors in ASD nuclear diagnosis, leading to unsuitable programs to facilitate their psycho- social and educative development. For this reason, it is necessary to encourage specific diagnostic scales based on specific cognitive- perceptive characteristics of neuropsychological information processing of people with ASD and not only behavioural criteria, in order to avoid common errors on ASD diagnostic.

Individuals with ASD are often diagnosed with widely symptom comorbidity associations. Over diagnostic multidivergence it is possible to find psychiatric comorbidities, including attention deficit, hyperactivity, emotions disorders, anxiety, schizotypal traits or severe depression (Lord, Elsabbagh, Baird & Veenstra-vanderweele, 2018), Moreover, other less studied conditions, such as post-traumatic stress it is currently broadening the symptomatic associations field (Kerns et al., 2020; Kildahl, Bakken & Iversen, 2019; Rumball, Happé & Grey, 2020).

As described by Golan, Haruvi-Lamdan, Laor & Horesh (2021), along their experimental investigations, they showed the presence of traumatic processes which had not been deeply studied by now reconsidered for analysis, as well as the inclusion of integrated response therapies for individuals with ASD.

Clinical associations, specifically, regarding epilepsy, constitutes the expression of specific neurological associations of ASD nuclear disorder, that courses with spontaneous and highly recurrent crisis. The estimated prevalence of this crisis is around 5-10/1000 of ASD specific individuals, although incidence may oscillate according to different countries (Amiet et al., 2013; Anukirthiga, Mishra, Pandey, Juneja & Sharma, 2019; Danielsson, Gillberg, Billstedt, Gillberg & Olsson 2005; Neumeyer et al., 2019), that exceed the percentages usual of normotypical group. As described by Liu et al. (2021) epilepsy prevalence is higher in adults with ASD than in children, which can point to a specific comorbid clinical condition of this disorder and both confuse itself. Therefore, the co-occurrence of health problems is significantly higher in people with ASD, which confers themselves vulnerability and an increased probability of presenting daily life skills development deficits (Lai et al., 2019). In this sense, Dickson, Galligan & Lok (2021) performed a relational study of different cognitive and intellectual abilities to analyze the recurrence of health-related clinical deficits and their relationship with individuals with ASD. Their study showed that the relationship of perceptual-cognitive skills, related to evidenced attention deficit and hyperactivity behaviours are significantly lower in people with ASD- compared to normotypical group. Moreover, as the degree of associated cognitive comorbidity level increases, it can make diagnosis harder (Brookman- Frazee et al., 2017).

According to Rosello et al. (2021) children with ASD showed severe deficits in attention with hyperactivity processes, leading to an evident nuclear diagnostic error. However, fundamental differences must be evaluated along cognitive flexibility-rigidity basic characteristic of ASD, in which, the differences found with high significance difference made through Wisconsin card test analysis (KWCST; Kado, Sanada, Oono, Ogino & Nouno, 2020). Meanwhile, attention disorder with hyperactivity presents almost the same symptoms that as ASD diagnosis, hence, the presence of severe components of attention deficits, impulsivity and hyperactivity, which lead to functional deficits, whose comorbidity association is very high, exceeding 10% in relation to ASD diagnosis (Casseus, 2022; Danielson et al., 2018).

More general symptoms, such as gastrointestinal disorder, constipation, digestion, among other clinical symptoms, have also been considered to be highly prevalent within ASD diagnosis, contributing greatly to the whole ASD symptoms (Bauman, 2010; Kohane et al., 2012). According to these studies, gastrointestinal disorders differ considerably regarding to sample heterogeneity studies of ASD type groups and normotypical group. Hence, Holingue, Poku, Pfeiffer, Murray & Fallin (2021) suggest that gastrointestinal deficits not only persist in an independent manner, but also significantly affect psycho-emotional processes and to the ability to fully participate along social- psychoeducational activities, such as curricular and extracurricular school tasks. Also, as a consequence of these disorders, important changes in diet are required as well as sleeping routines and other general medical conditions.

The strong genetic basis of ASD and its multiple genetic combinations, which affects the neuropsychological component of information processing, may be based on the relationship between comorbid symptomatic variability on individuals with ASD, which requires special attention if we want to perform programs properly adapted to basic nuclear needs of these people. Indeed, Hellquist & Tanmmimies (2021), just like Chiarotti & Venerosi (2020) and Lord et al. (2020) corroborate this strong genetic basis along diagnosis of ASD, whose estimated prevalence stands on 1/160 of children born, showing some variability between demographic studies.

Schaefer et al. (2013) carried out studies showing the presence of selected genes loci on specific genome that characterizes ASD people; however, the information regarding genetic studies in early childhood were still very limited. In their study accomplished with 868 families and 213 adolescents and adults with ASD, only 9.1% of families and 2.8% of adolescents and adults with ASD had been referred for genetic analysis. And, of those who had been derived, significant genetic etiological relationships were found ($p< .001$), with significant levels of associated neurodevelopmental deficits ($p< .01$), including cognitive impairment ($p< .001$) and/or a specific language disorder ($p< .001$) about.

This research has two fundamental **general aims**: 1) to analyse the significance levels of comorbidity symptoms associated with nuclear diagnosis of people with ASD, and, above all, 2) to verify if there were differences between the comorbidity symptomatic groups found between normotypical and ASD groups, and, consequently proving that the comorbidity associated processes are specific and differential regarding ASD symptoms.

Method

Research design

Research design is based on the design of an ad hoc questionnaire, which includes questions related to all symptomatic factors empirically refuted through previous investigation studies. Questionnaire analysed continuous quantitative ordinal values and other complementary qualitative values. Data for continuous quantitative variables was analyzed throughout post-hoc multivariate test regarding selected fixed variables: group, age and sex, valued with SPSS statistical set. Qualitative values complement to previous ones.

Participants

A total of 390 participants joined this study, of which the experimental group was composed by the three ASD′ diagnosis levels (n: 262) and one control group of 128 normotypical participants, whose distribution according to group type, age ranges and sex can be seen in **Table 1**. The sample consisted mainly of participants from Spain and South America.

Table 1. Participants Group * Age * Sex (N= 390).

Sex			*Age*					*Total*
			2.0-5.9 yo	6.0- 9.9 yo	10.0-13.9 yo	14.0-17.9 yo	>18.0 yo	2-5.9
Man	Group	TYPICAL	13	24	21	3	2	63
		ASD-1	36	30	18	12	13	109
		ASD-2	20	19	13	7	10	69
		ASD-3	16	14	4	2	7	43
	Total		85	87	56	24	32	284
Woman	Group	TYPICAL	15	19	5	3	23	65
		ASD-1	0	1	5	2	7	15
		ASD-2	6	3	2	2	1	14
		ASD-3	2	4	0	1	5	12
	Total		23	27	12	8	36	106
TOTAL								**390**

Variables

A total of 3 fixed variables were selected: 1) Group made of a normotypical group and three experimental groups: ASD-1, ASD-2 and ASD-3 groups, 2) Age composed by 5 age intervals: 2- 5.9 yo, 6- 9.9 yo, 10 - 13.9 yo, 15-17-9 yo, and >18 yo, and 3) Two groups related to sex variable: male and female.

A total of 25 dynamic variables were analysed to verify the presence of comorbid symptom groups associated to ASD diagnosis: 1) attention, 2) memory, 3) intellectual capacity, 4) hyperactivity, 5) behavioural disorders, 6) schizotypal traits, 7) anxiety, 8) depression, 9) emotional stress, 10) sleep problems, 11) linguistic development, 12) dyslalias- dysarthrias of language, 13) developmental, 14) movement dynamics, 15) visuo-motor coordination, 16) epilepsy, 17) cancer symptoms, 18) cardiological disease, 19) respiratory affection, 20) diabetes, 32) allergies, 22) intestinal constipation, 23) digestion, 24) vision, and 25) hearing.

Variables were grouped into dimensions based on previous empirical studies, through statistical calculation of transform-calculate variables, we obtained seven specific dimensions for statistical evaluation: I) **Cognition**, integrated of attention, memory and intellectual ability variables, II) **Behavioral**, composed by the following variables: hyperactivity, behavioural disorders, anxiety, emotional stress and sleep deficits, III) **Psychoaffective,** which include schizotypal traits and depressive processes variables, IV) **Specific- clinic**, composed by following variables: epilepsy and allergies, V) **General- clinic**, integrated by cancer symptoms, cardiological affection, respiratory affection, diabetes, intestinal constipation, digestion, vision and hearing variables, VI) **Language**, calculated by mean in linguistic development and presence of dyslalia and dysarthria disorders, and VII) **Psychomotor**, which include maturational development, movement dynamic and visuomotor coordination.

Results

Reliability study

Sample reliability selected sample calculated by means of Cronbach's Alpha analysis for all the study items, which included both variables and calculated dimensions (items: 36). Level α: .908, which shows a high reliability and validity rightly to goals of this study.

General multivariate test

This analysis shows the main effects of dimensions calculated from 25 dynamic variables on fixed isolated variables and their intersection. Results can be observed in **Table 2**.

Table 2. Multivariate test main effects.

Effect	Stat.	Value	F	Hypot.	Error	Sig.	Eta	Noncent. Parameter	Observed Power
Intercept	**Pillai's Trace**	.91	560.76	7.00	346.00	.00	.91	3925.38	1.00
Group		.34	6.35	21.00	104.00	.00	.11	133.47	1.00
Age		.15	1.99	28.00	1396.00	.00	.03	55.92	.99
Sex		.15	1.99	28.00	1396.00	.00	.03	55.92	.99
*Group*Age*		.33	1.44	84.00	2464.00	.00	.04	12.,75	1.00
Group Sex*		.07	1.34	21.00	1044.00	.14	.02	28.13	.91
*Group*Age*Sex*		.22	1.14	70.00	2464.00	.20	.03	79.84	.99

Multivariate Pillai's Trace statistical analysis to effects of seven dimensions over three fixed variables, showed significant critical level of variables intersection as well as isolated variables analysis (sig: .00, F: 560.76), showing significant differences in the calculated dimensions over fixed variables intersection: group, age and sex. Likewise, when the effects of these dimensions are analysed one by one, data also show differential critical level, being the dimensions′ effects over the group variable (sig: .00), age (sig: .00) and sex (sig: .00).

However, when both variables are correlated, critical levels effects of study dimensions are scattered, being group variable with sex (sig: .00), but other multiple correlation no longer offer differential critical levels: group* sex: sig: 14, and group* age* sex: sig:.20.

Comparative analysis to group variable

The main aim of this study is to analyse if there are differences between the effects of the calculated dimensions regarding to group type, and, above all, regarding to normotypical group and experimental group (three ASD levels).

Comparative analysis performed for seven dimensions calculated from analysis to group variable was performed through the Tukey or Games-Howell post-hoc test, according Levene′s index previously found.

Levene′s test index for variances equality found was significant for all dimensions (<.05), but not regarding cognition dimension (.62). For this reason, cognition dimension was analysed with Games-Howell statistic- test, while other study dimensions were analysed with Tukey statistic.

Table 3 shows the conclusive comparative data.

Table 3. Multivariate Test Post-hoc to Group variable.

DV: DIMENSIONS	Group (post-hoc)		µ difference	Std. error	Sig. (95%)
COGNITION	TYPICAL	ASD1	-1.83(*)	.26	.00
		ASD2	-3.07(*)	.28	.00
		ASD3	-3.89(*)	.35	.00
	ASD1	ASD2	-1.24(*)	.29	.00
		ASD3	-2.05(*)	.33	.00
	ASD2	ASD3	-.81 (*)	.35	.10
BEHAVIOURAL	TYPICAL	ASD1	-4.26	.46	.00
		ASD2	-4.70	.52	.00
		ASD3	-6.25	.59	.00
	ASD1	ASD2	-.42	.52	.84
		ASD3	-1.98	.59	.00
	ASD2	ASD3	-1.55	.64	.07
PSYCHOAFFECTIVE	TYPICAL	ASD1	-.80	.16	.00
		ASD2	-.88	.18	.00
		ASD3	-1.23	.21	.00
	ASD1	ASD2	-.07	.18	.97
		ASD3	-.42	.21	.18
	ASD2	ASD3	-.35	.22	.42
SPECIFIC- CLINIC	TYPICAL	ASD1	-.22	.11	.20
		ASD2	-.25	.12	.19
		ASD3	-.45	.14	.01
	ASD1	ASD2	-.03	.12	.99
		ASD3	-.22	.14	.40
	ASD2	ASD3	-.19	.15	.59
GENERAL-CLINIC	TYPICAL	ASD1	-.39	.28	.51
		ASD2	-.43	.32	.52
		ASD3	-.61	.36	.34
	ASD1	ASD2	-.04	.32	.99
		ASD3	-.21	.37	.93
	ASD2	ASD3	-.17	.39	.97
LANGUAGE	TYPICAL	ASD1	-1.98	.33	.00
		ASD2	-3.69	.36	.00
		ASD3	-5.68	.42	.00
	ASD1	ASD2	-1.71	.37	.00
		ASD3	-3.70	.42	.00
	ASD2	ASD3	-1.98	.45	.00
PSYCHOMOTOR	TYPICAL	ASD1	-1.75	,21	,00
		ASD2	-2.66	,24	,00
		ASD3	-3.15	,27	,00
	ASD1	ASD2	-.91	,24	,00
		ASD3	-1.39	,28	,00
	ASD2	ASD3	-.48	,33	,47

(*) Games- Howell.

These results show significant differences in cognition dimension between the experimental group (ASD-1-2-3) and normotypical control group. Likewise, there are also significant differences between ASD-1 level group and ASD2 and ASD 3 level groups; however, no significant differences were found between ASD-2 and ASD-3 level groups (sig: .07). Visual dispersion of data for cognition dimension can be observed graphically in diagram (see **Figure 1**).

Figure 1. Cognition plot.

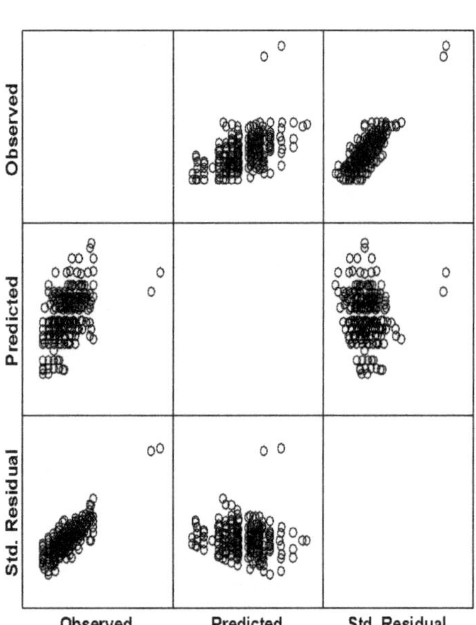

Behaviour dimension also presents significant differences between normotypical group and experimental groups. However, data between several experimental group levels are different, thus, differential levels between the ASD-1 and ASD-3 groups are observed, but no differences between ASD-1 and ASD-2 (sig: .84) are found, either, significant differences between the ASD-2 and 3 group are found (sig: .07).

Visual dispersion levels can be seen in **Figure 2**.

Figure 2. Behavioural plot.

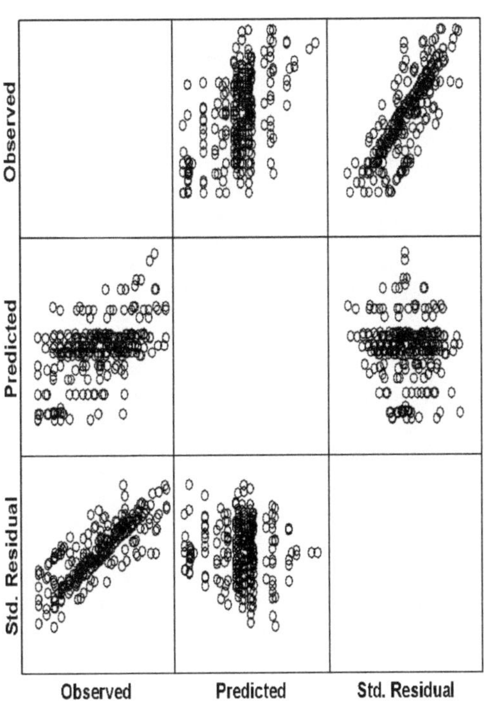

Regarding to psychoaffective dimension, significant differences were observed between the normotypical control group and the experimental groups. However, no significant critical levels were found between the different ASD group levels.

Graphic dispersion of measurements can be seen in Figure 3.

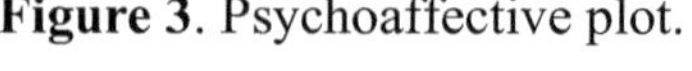

Figure 3. Psychoaffective plot.

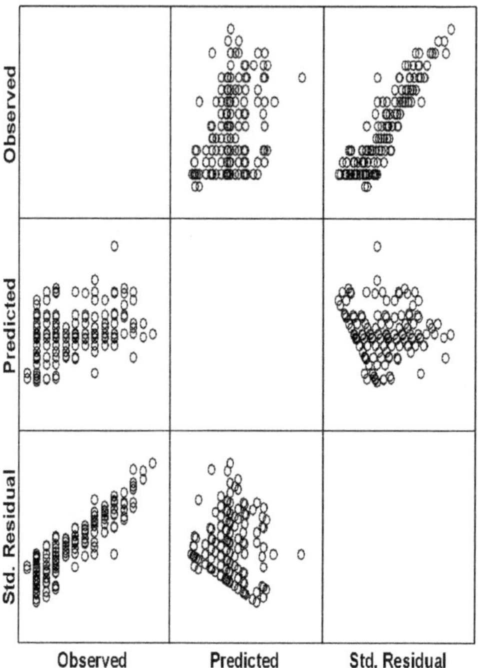

Also, in specific- clinical dimension, data show significant differences between normotypical control group regarding to ASD-3 level group (sig: .01); but no significant differences were found between the normotypical group regarding to ASD-1 and ASD- 2 group, neither between the three ASD levels of experimental group.

Figure 4 shows the graphical dispersion.

Figure 4. Specific- clinic plot.

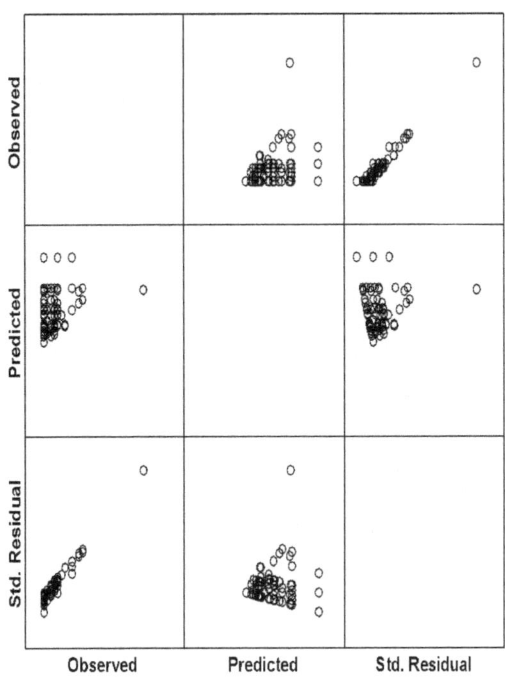

In order to gen mor insight into the comorbidity of epilepsy and ASD diagnosis an analysis isolated variable dimension′ was carried out: epilepsy and allergies.

According to previous Levene′s significant index, data through Tukey's test is shown in Table 4.

Table 4. Multivariate test para epilepsy and allergies (specific-clinic dimension).

DV	*Group (post-hoc)*		*μ difference*	*Std. error*	*Sig. (95%)*
Epilepsy	typical	ASD1	-.15	.08	.22
		ASD2	-.08	.08	.75
		ASD3	-.40(*)	.10	.00
	ASD1	ASD2	.06	.09	.89
		ASD3	-.25	.10	.07
	ASD2	ASD3	-.31	.15	.17
Allergies	typical	ASD1	-.13	.15	.80
		ASD2	-.33	.16	.20
		ASD3	-.09	.19	.96
	ASD1	ASD2	-.19	.16	.66
		ASD3	.04	.19	.99
	ASD2	ASD3	.23	.20	.66

Indeed, results indicate a significant critical level for epilepsy variable between the normotypic group and ASD-3 experimental group (sig: .00), however, no significant differences between normotypic group and the ASD-1-2 groups are found. Neither significant difference between the three levels of experimental groups were found.

On allergy variable no significant differences between groups were found.

Complementary qualitative analysis pointed out that allergies variable co- occurs according to the following frequencies with: acarus (37), lactose (14), pollen (12), grasses (10), various foods (9), gluten (7), egg (6), humidity (6), dermatitis (6), fructose (5), wool (5), rhinitis (4), cold (3), dog hair (3), oxcarbazepine (2) , sun (2), ampicillin (2), insect bites (2), ibuprofen (2), tomato (2), cephalexin (2), celiac disease (1), amoxicillin (1), asthma (1). However, allergic variable was found indistinctly in normotypical control group and ASD experimental groups.

General-clinical dimension showed no differences between studied groups. However, some exceptions stand out. Thus, cardiovascular variable showed significant differences between the normotypical group and ASD-1 group (sig: .01) and ASD-2 group (sig: .04); as well as, audition variable where- significant were observed between the ASD-2 and ASD-3 groups (sig: .02). Graphic dispersion data can be seen in Figure 5.

Figure 5. general- clinic plot.

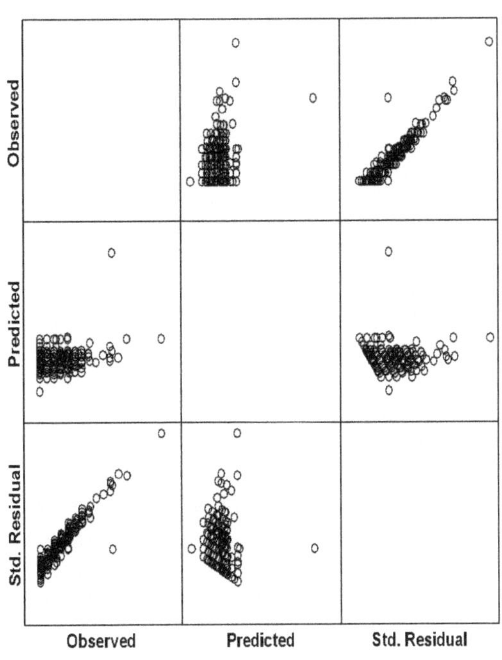

Regarding to language dimension, differences were- significant between normotypical group and experimental level groups, as well as between the three of experimental group levels itself, whose graphical dispersion data can be seen in Figure 6.

Figure 6. Language plot.

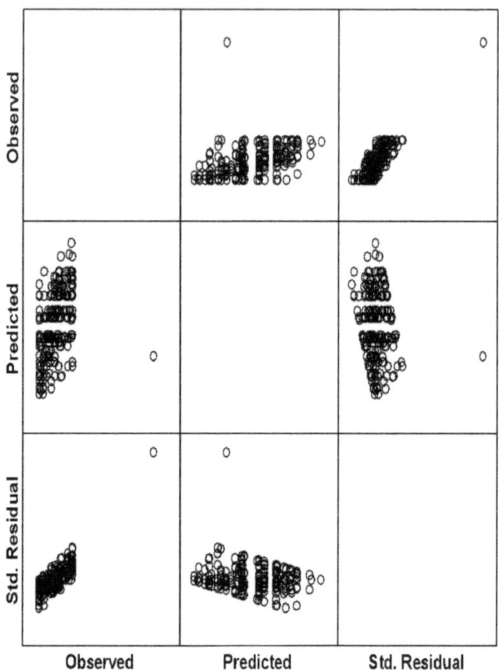

Finally, regarding to psychomotor dimension, there were also significant differences between the normotypical group and the three experimental group levels of, as well as between all the experimental group levels of, but no significant differences were found between ASD-2 and ASD-3 groups found (sig: .47) (see **Figure 7**).

Figure 7. Psychomotor plot.

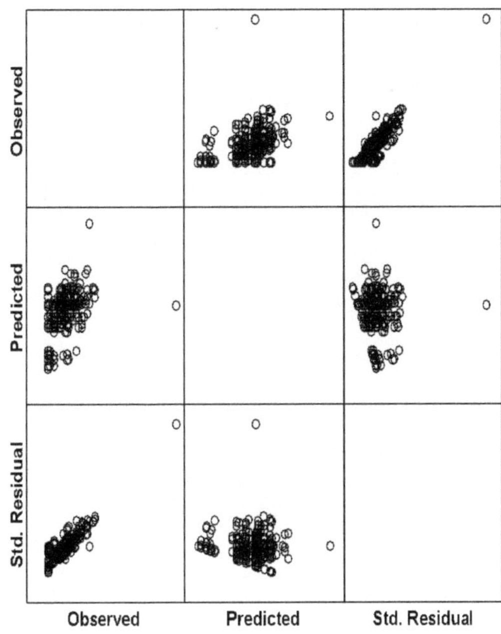

Discussion

Making a nuclear basis diagnosis that differs from other symptom associated groups like comorbidity it is required in order to avoid errors caused by very subtle differences in symptomatology. This problem could be solved by performing specific genetic and genomic analysis ASDs diagnosed people.

In this sense, the performance of genetic analysis has been recommended by several medical societies (Schaefer & Mendelsohn, 2013). Furthermore, previous studies pointed to an important role of genetic background in the ASD symptomatology as it has been shown for the Fragile X syndrome (Moeschler et al., 2014), as well as the copy number variant (CNV) screens throughout chromosomal microarrays (CMA) (Miller et al., 2010; Schaefer et al., 2013).

Furthermore, recent publications suggest that whole exome sequencing (WES) should be used as diagnostic first-level CGT for people with ASD (Srivastava et al., 2019). The American College of Medical Genetics and Genomics (ACMG) also recommended that WES or whole genome sequencing (WGS) should be considered aa an essential tool for diagnosis in children with congenital cluster, developmentally delayed or intellectual disability.

It has been published by Tammimies et al (2015) that this kind of genetic analysis were positive in 8-15% of people with ASD evaluated, and between 8-25% regarding WES performance.

In summary, limitations of ASD diagnosis could lead to errors, therefore it is necessary to empirically verify and improve diagnosis in order to differentiate the nuclear disorder from the associated comorbidities symptom. Moreover, new strategies are required to optimize the identification and early intervention for all children suspected of having ASD + other comorbidities diagnosis about.

In this sense, Ojea (2022) has developed a scale for integrated analysis of criteria behaviours indicated by DSM-5 classification and the particularities of information cognitive- perceptive processing coding in people with ASD. Scale analyses the variants of perceptual and encoding processing, as well as the development of relationships between information systems (input- output) and the type of information retrieval from permanent semantic memory. Hence, it is possible integrate the behavioural basic components with interrelated neuronal- relationships values to clarify the ASD′ nuclear diagnosis. Subsequently, any comorbid association could be included within the main diagnosis ones.

Therefore, formative consideration of ASD basic nuclear diagnosis constitutes only a profile of didactic programmatic implementation, which, it will be adapted to diagnosed symptomatic comorbid groups. Thus, diagnosis as a whole will go from individual specific psychoeducational needs, in which, comorbidity symptoms must start from particular coding- processing way of ASD′, to a nuclear diagnosis like the main diagnostic.

Specific behavioural or rehabilitation therapies must support the specific nuclear processing itself. For now, many indications or applied therapies are not effective for the improvement of people with ASD. Indeed, this particular processing way of ASD people means that many indications are not well perceived or understood by individuals with ASD, being a big handicap in the therapy process. This is something that should be prioritised when it comes to the development of a therapy strategy.

Conclusion

In this study, we shown that ASD′ diagnosis is associated with several comorbid symptomatic groups, regarding to the following dimensions: cognition, behaviour, psychoaffective alterations and specific- clinical symptoms. It should be noted the relevance of variables such as epilepsy variable, language alterations and psychomotor deficits. Some comorbidity presents a very high frequency and intensity, e.g., psychoaffective disorders, specially, regarding to schizotypal traits, anxiety or depression. Descriptive statistics related to behaviour are also noteworthy, specially, those regarding attention, attention deficit- hyperactivity disorder, emotional disorders and language specific deficits, which showed very high levels comorbidity with ASD diagnosis. However, no specific differences between different selected groups were found regarding to general- clinical. These intensity levels on comorbidity symptoms can lead to initial errors on ASD nuclear specific diagnosis, leading to a wrong specific diagnosis of attention deficit or attention and hyperactivity deficit with impulsivity diagnosis.

Indeed, due to this observation the specific intervention process can also be erroneous, leading to a loss of essential time that could be invested in an integral socio- personal development. This fact is very important, because if it´s like this, specific intervention consequent process also can be erroneous and lose essential time for socio- personal integral development.

For this reason, diagnosis should not be based jus on analysis of observable behaviours, but also on the analysis of highly specific factors and dimensions regarding specific conditions derived from genetic groups. In this sense, the influence on neuronal synapses regarding information processing fluidity, which is severely affected in people with ASD must be also analysed. Specific processing shows a very particular way of information coding specifically differentiates it from other specific diagnose groups. Hence, it could possible avoid the current diagnostic errors on diagnosis.

Depending on how accurate the ASD diagnosis is, it can be possible to determine the associated comorbid variants, which are underlying the secondary diagnostic process.

Therefore, it is required to develop an integrated diagnostic system, which is effective and valid. Moreover, a multivariable program based on this data must be developed in order to improve specific coding-processing and comorbidity symptoms associated to ASD.

References

American Psychiatric Association. (2013). *Diagnostic and Statistical Manual of Mental Disorders- DSM-5* (5th ed.). American Psychiatric Publishin. https://www.psychiatry.org/psychiatrists/practice/dsm

Amiet, C., Gourfinkel-An, I., Laurent, C., Carayol, J. R., Génin, B. R., Leguern, E., Tordjman, S., & Cohen, D. (2013). Epilepsy in simplex autism pedigrees is much lower than the rate in multiplex autism pedigrees. *Biological Psychiatry, 74*(3). e3-e4. DOI: 10.1016/j.biopsych.2013.01.037

Anukirthiga, B., Mishra, D., Pandey, S., Juneja, M., & Sharma, N. (2019). Prevalence of epilepsy and interictal epileptiform discharges in children with autism and attention-deficit hyperactivity disorder. *Indian Journal of Pediatrics, 86*, 897-902. https://doi.org/10.1007/s12098-019-02977-6

Bauman, M. L. (2010). Medical comorbidities in autism: Challenges to diagnosis and treatment. *Neurotherapeutics, 7*(3), 320- 327. https://doi.org/10.1016/j.nurt.2010.06.001

Brookman-Frazee, L., Stadnick, N., Chlebowski, C., Baker- Ericzén, M. J., & Ganger, W. (2017). Characterizing psychiatric comorbidity in children with autism spectrum disorder receiving publicly funded mental health services. *Autism, 22*(8), 938- 952. https://doi.org/10.1177/1362361317712650

Casseus, M. (2022). Prevalence of co-occurring autism spectrum disorder and attention deficit/hyperactivity disorder among children in the United States. *Autism, 26*(6) 159-1597. DOI: 10.1177/13623613221083279

Chiarotti, F., & Venerosi, A. (2020). Epidemiology of autism spectrum disorders: A review of worldwide prevalence estimates since 2014. *Brain Sciences, 10*(5). E274. https://doi.org/10.3390/brainsci10050274

Danielson, M. L., Bitsko, R. H., Ghandour, R. M., Holbrook, J. R., Kogan, M. D., & Blumberg, S. J. (2018). Prevalence of parent-reported ADHD diagnosis and associated treatment among U.S. children and adolescents, 2016. *Journal of Clinical Child and Adolescent Psychology, 47*(2), 199- 212. https://doi.org/10.1080/15374416.2017.1417860

Danielsson, S., Gillberg, I. C., Billstedt, E., Gillberg, C., & Olsson, I. (2005). Epilepsy in young adults with autism: A prospective population-based follow-up study of 120 individuals diagnosed in childhood. *Epilepsia, 46*(6), 918- 923. https://doi.org/10.1111/j.1528-1167.2005.57504.x

Dickson, K. S., Galligan, M. L., & Lok, H. (2021). Short report: A quantitative methodological review of participant characteristics in the literature testing mental health interventions for youth with autism spectrum disorder. *Autism, 26*(4) 995-1000 DOI: 10.1177/13623613211056408

Golan, O., Haruvi-Lamdan, N., Laor, N., & Horesh, D. (2021). The comorbidity between autism spectrum disorder and post-traumatic stress disorder is mediated by brooding rumination. *Autism, 26*(2) 538-544. DOI: 10.1177/13623613211035240

Hellquist, A., & Tammimies, K. (2021). Access, utilization, and awareness for clinical genetic testing in autism spectrum disorder in Sweden: A survey study. *Autism, 26*(7) 1795- 1804. DOI: 10.1177/13623613211066130

Holingue, C., Poku, O., Pfeiffer, D., Murray, S., & Fallin, D. (2021). Gastrointestinal concerns in children with autism spectrum disorder: A qualitative study of family experiences. *Autism, 26*(7) 1698- 1711. DOI: 10.1177/13623613211062667

Kado, Y., Sanada, S., Oono, S., Ogino, T., & Nouno, S. (2020). Children with autism spectrum disorder comorbid with attention-deficit/hyperactivity disorder examined by the Wisconsin card sorting test: Analysis by age-related differences. *Brain Development, 42*, 113- 120

Kerns, C. M., Berkowitz, S. J., Moskowitz, L. J., Drahota, A., Lerner, M. D., & Newschaffer, C. J. (2020). Screening and treatment of trauma-related symptoms in youth with autism spectrum disorder among community providers in the United States. *Autism, 24*(2), 515- 525. https://doi. org/10.1177/13623613 19847908

Kildahl, A. N., Bakken, T. L., & Iversen, T. E. (2019). Identification of post-traumatic stress disorder in individuals with autism spectrum disorder and intellectual disability: A systematic review identification of post-traumatic stress disorder in individuals with autism spectrum disorder and intellectual. *Journal of Mental Health Research in Intellectual Disabilities, 12*(1- 2), 1- 25. https://doi.org/10.1 080/19315864.2019.1595233

Kohane, I. S., McMurry, A., Weber, G., MacFadden, D., Rappaport, L., Kunkel, L., Bickel, J., Wattanasin, N., Spence, S., & Murphy, S. (2012). The co-morbidity burden of children and young adults with autism spectrum disorders. *PLOS ONE, 7*(4). e33224. https://doi. org/10.1371/journal.pone.0033224

Lai, M.-C., Kassee, C., Besney, R., Bonato, S., Hull, L., Mandy, W., Szatmari, P., & Ameis, S. H. (2019). Prevalence of co-occurring mental health diagnoses in the autism population: A systematic review and meta-analysis. *The Lancet Psychiatry, 6*(10), 819- 829. https://doi.org/10.1016/s2215-0366(19)30289-5

Liu, X., Sun, X, Sun, C., Zou, M., Chen, Y., Huang, J., Wu, L., & Chen, W. (2021). Prevalence of epilepsy in autism spectrum disorders: A systematic review and meta-analysis. *Autism, 26*(1) 33- 50. DOI: 10.1177/13623613211045029

Lord, C., Elsabbagh, M., Baird, G., & Veenstra- vanderweele, J. (2018). Autism spectrum disorder. *The Lancet, 392*, 508- 520. https://doi.org/10.1016/S0140-6736(18)31129-2

Miller, D. T., Adam, M. P., Aradhya, S., Biesecker, L. G., Brothman, A. R., Carter, N. … & Ledbetter, D. H. (2010). Consensus statement: Chromosomal microarray is a first-tier clinical diagnostic test for individuals with developmental disabilities or congenital anomalies. *American Journal of Human Genetics, 86*(5), 749- 764. https://doi.org/10.1016/j.ajhg.2010.04.006

Moeschler, J. B., Shevell, M., & Committee on Genetics. (2014). Comprehensive evaluation of the child with intellectual disability or global developmental delays. *Pediatrics, 134*(3), e903- e918. https://doi.org/10.1542/peds.2014-1839

Neumeyer, A. M., Anixt, J., Chan, J., Perrin, J. M., Murray, D., Coury, D. L., Bennett, A., Farmer, J., & Parker, R. A. (2019). Identifying associations among co-occurring medical conditions in children with autism spectrum disorders. *Academic Pediatrics, 19*(3), 300- 306. https://doi. org/10.1016/j.acap.2018.06.014

Ojea, M. (2021). Classification of the comorbid symptomatic groups on Autism Spectrum Disorder diagnosis. *International Journal for Innovation Education and Research, 9*(6), 196- 208. ISSN: 2411- 293301. https://scholarsjournal.net/index.php/ijier/issue/view/94

Ojea, M. (2022). Integrated Scale for Diagnosis of Autism Spectrum Disorder (ISD-ASD). *International Journal for Innovation, Education and Research, 10*(9), 202-274. https://scholarsjournal.net/index.php/ijier/article/view/3906/2659

Rosello, R., Martinez-Raga, J., Mira, A., Pastor, J. C., Solmi, M., & Cortese, S. (2021). Cognitive, social, and behavioral manifestations of the co-occurrence of autism spectrum disorder and attention-deficit/hyperactivity disorder: A systematic review. *Autism, 26*(4) 743- 760. DOI: 10.1177/13623613211065545

Rumball, F., Happé, F., & Grey, N. (2020). Experience of trauma and PTSD symptoms in autistic adults: Risk of PTSD development following DSM-5 and non-DSM-5 traumatic life events. *Autism Research, 13*(12), 2122- 2132. https://doi.org/10.1002/aur.2306

Schaefer, G. B., Mendelsohn, N. J., & Professional Practice Guidelines Committee. (2013). Clinical genetics evaluation in identifying the etiology of autism spectrum disorders: 2013 guideline revisions. *Genetics in Medicine, 15*(5), 399-407. https://doi.org/10.1038/gim.2013.32

Srivastava, S., Love-Nichols, J. A., Dies, K. A., Ledbetter, D. H., Martin, C. L., Chung, W. K., Firth, H. V., Frazier, T., Hansen, R. L., Prock, L., Brunner, H., Hoang, N., Scherer, S. W., Sahin, M., Miller, D. T., & NDD Exome Scoping Review Work Group. (2019). Meta-analysis and multidisciplinary consensus statement: Exome sequencing is a firsttier clinical diagnostic test for individuals with neurodevelopmental disorders. *Genetics in Medicine, 21*(11), 2413- 2421. https://doi.org/10.1038/s41436-019-0554-6

Tammimies, K., Marshall, C. R., Walker, S., Kaur, G., Thiruvahindrapuram, B., Lionel, A. C. . . . & Fernandez, B. A. (2015). Molecular diagnostic yield of chromosomal microarray analysis and whole-exome sequencing in children with autism spectrum disorder. *JAMA, 314*(9), 895- 903. https://doi.org/10.1001/jama.2015.10078

www.ingramcontent.com/pod-product-compliance
Lightning Source LLC
LaVergne TN
LVHW021312160826

845679LV00001B/323
* 9 7 9 8 8 9 2 4 8 4 5 0 3 *